BODYBUILDING WORKOUT PLAN FOR BEGINNERS

Using An Effective Roadmap To Unlock Your Potential

ROBERT CARGILL

TABLE OF CONTENTS

EXERCISE IS IMPORTANT

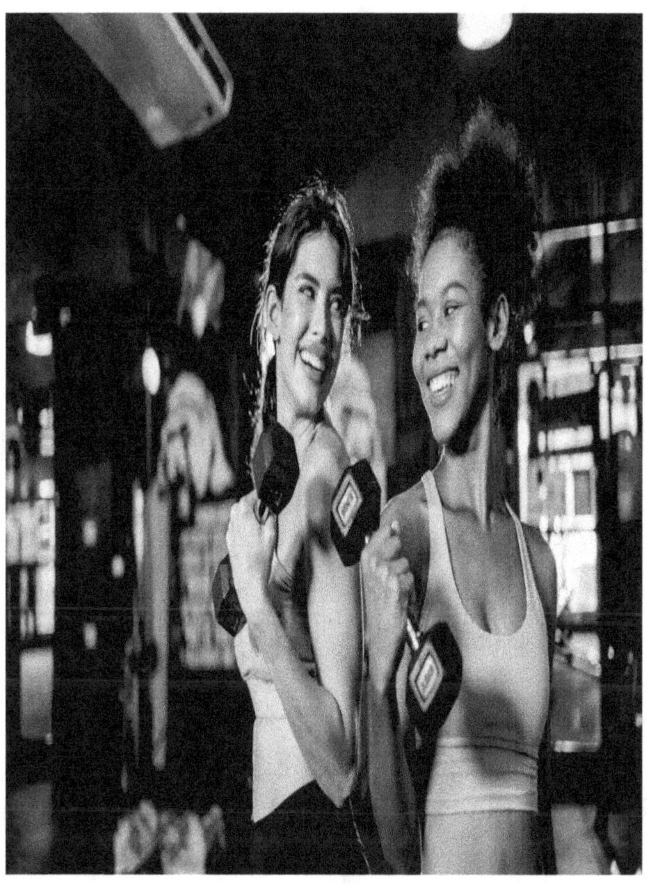

INTRODUCTION

Welcome to the world of bodybuilding, where strength, discipline, and dedication join together to create a body that exudes power and confidence. Whether you want to create an ideal muscular physique or simply live a healthier, more active lifestyle, this book, "Bodybuilding Workout Plan for Beginners," is your thorough guide to getting started on a revolutionary journey. In these pages, we will walk you through each stage of your bodybuilding journey, providing you with the knowledge, ideas, and practical training routines you need to get started. This book is designed specifically for beginners, people who have just begun their fitness adventure, or those attempting to transition into the bodybuilding field. Regardless of your current level of fitness or understanding of the gym, this comprehensive book will teach you all you need to know to maximize your potential.

We understand that beginning a bodybuilding routine may be overwhelming, with so many workouts, food plans, and contradictory advise. That is why we have simplified the complex world of bodybuilding into a concise and easy-to-understand handbook designed specifically for beginners like you. By following the professional advice and tried-and-true training routines outlined in this book, you will lay a solid foundation for your bodybuilding goals and set yourself up for long-term success. We will go into the fundamental concepts of bodybuilding in the pages that follow, addressing topics such as nutrition, workout selection, proper form, and the need of rest and recuperation. We will guide you through an intelligently designed training plan that targets all major muscle groups, ensuring balanced growth and lowering your risk of injury. Furthermore, we will explore common difficulties encountered by newcomers and give practical solutions to overcome them, keeping you motivated and focused on your goals.

Remember that bodybuilding is more than just physical transformation; it is an attitude and a way of life that fosters self-discipline, determination, and persistence. The journey may not always be easy, but with the right information, guidance, and unwavering dedication, you may achieve incredible results.

CHAPTER 1. Bodybuilding Fundamentals

What exactly is bodybuilding?

Bodybuilding is a type of physical exercise that entails intense training and muscular development through resistance activities like weightlifting. It is a sport that focuses on sculpting and shaping the body in order to develop a muscular and appealing physique. Bodybuilders work out hard and live a disciplined lifestyle in order to enhance muscle growth and reduce body fat.

Bodybuilding Advantages

Bodybuilding has numerous advantages beyond simply increasing muscular mass. To begin with, it increases overall physical strength and endurance, making daily chores easier to do. Weight exercise on a regular basis increases bone density and lowers the risk of osteoporosis. Bodybuilding also improves cardiovascular health and can help lower blood pressure.

Another big benefit of bodybuilding is its favorable effect on mental health. The discipline required for exercise and eating a healthy diet builds confidence and self-control. Setting and accomplishing bodybuilding objectives can increase self-esteem and create a sense of success. Furthermore, exercise releases endorphins, which are natural mood-enhancing substances, resulting in less stress and better mental health.

Establishing Realistic Goals

Setting realistic goals in bodybuilding is critical for ensuring success and avoiding potential setbacks. It is critical to set achievable short-term and long-term goals that are matched to individual capabilities. Realistic objectives may include increasing muscle mass, decreasing body fat percentage, or boosting strength in specific workouts.

Setting realistic goals requires taking into account aspects such as age, current fitness level, and genetic predispositions. Consultation with a fitness professional or personal trainer can provide helpful guidance in establishing appropriate goals and planning an effective training program.

Bodybuilding and Nutrition

Nutrition is critical in bodybuilding since it has a direct impact on muscle growth, recuperation, and overall performance. A well-balanced diet rich in protein, carbs, and healthy fats is crucial for addressing the increased energy demands of strenuous activities. Protein is very vital in bodybuilding since it serves as the foundation for muscle repair and growth. High-quality protein sources, such as lean meats, fish, eggs, and lentils, should be included in meals. Carbohydrates fuel workouts and replenish glycogen stores, while healthy fats promote hormone production and joint health.

Bodybuilders should consider micronutrients such as vitamins and minerals in addition to macronutrients. These nutrients are necessary for a variety of biological processes as well as general wellness. Proper hydration is also essential for muscular function and recovery. Bodybuilders frequently follow specialized dietary programs to maximize nutrition, such as tracking macronutrient ratios or taking supplements such as protein powders or vitamins. However, it is best to work with a qualified dietitian or nutritionist to create a dietary plan that is tailored to your specific needs and goals.

Finally, bodybuilding is a multifaceted approach to physical training and muscle development. It has several advantages, including increased strength, cardiovascular health, and mental well-being.

Setting realistic goals and adhering to a balanced diet plan are critical components of bodybuilding success and living a healthy lifestyle.

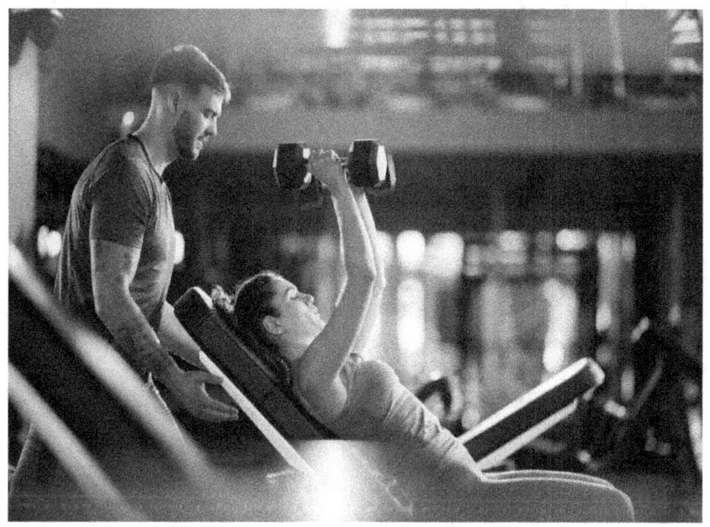

CHAPTER 2. How to Begin Your Fitness Journey

Evaluate Your Current Fitness Level

Beginning a fitness journey requires an honest evaluation of your present fitness level. Take a minute to assess your own strengths and shortcomings, as well as your general health. Think about your endurance, flexibility, and strength. This self-evaluation will assist you in setting realistic objectives and tailoring your exercises to your individual requirements.

Making a Workout Schedule

When it comes to reaching fitness objectives, consistency is essential. Developing an exercise routine that matches your lifestyle is critical for long-term success. Determine how many days a week you can devote to exercising and schedule your routines accordingly. Establishing a pattern, whether it's early in the morning, during lunch breaks, or in the evenings, can help you remain on track and make exercise a regular part of your life.

Selecting the Best Gym or Home Setup

The choice between a gym membership and a home training setting is determined by your tastes, available resources, and available space. A gym may be the best option if you thrive in a social setting, love group classes, or require access to specific equipment. If convenience, privacy, and flexibility are essential to you, putting up a home gym with simple equipment may be a good alternative. When making this option, keep your money, convenience, and personal preferences in mind.

Required Equipment for Beginners

Beginners should start with a few crucial pieces of equipment that will help them achieve a well-rounded exercise. These necessities are as follows:

- **Invest in breathable and flexible training:** Apparel that allows for effortless movement and wicks away perspiration.
- **Proper footwear:** Select sports shoes that give enough support, cushioning, and stability for the activities you want to participate in.

- **Non-slip exercise mats:** Provide a cushioned surface for floor workouts, stretching, and core work.
- **Resistance bands:** These adaptable bands come in a range of resistance levels and may be used for strength training routines that target specific muscle regions.
- **Dumbbells or kettlebells:** To include strength training into your regimen, begin with a set of low to moderate weights.
- **Jump rope:** Is a low-cost cardio item that may be used both indoors and outdoors to increase heart rate and coordination.

Remember that as a novice, simplicity is essential. Concentrate on learning the fundamentals first, then progressively increasing the intensity and intricacy of your exercises as you develop. To guarantee appropriate form and technique, seek advice from fitness professionals, trainers, or trusted internet resources. You are well on your way to reaching your fitness objectives and adopting a healthy lifestyle if you are dedicated, consistent, and have the correct mentality.

CHAPTER 3. Weight Training Fundamentals

Recognizing the Different Types of Exercises

Weight training is a very effective kind of exercise that may help people gain strength, muscular mass, and general fitness. To get the most out of weight training, you must first grasp the various types of exercises. Compound exercises are movements that work numerous muscle groups at the same time. These exercises are great for increasing general strength and encouraging functional motions.

Isolation exercises, on the other hand, concentrate on a single muscle group. Common isolation workouts include bicep curls, tricep extensions, and calf raises. These exercises can be beneficial for addressing certain muscular imbalances or developing specific muscles.

Appropriate Form and Technique

Maintaining good form and technique is one of the most important parts of weight training. It not only increases the exercise's efficacy but also reduces the chance of damage. When doing weightlifting workouts, it is critical to:

- Throughout the activity, keep a neutral spine and appropriate posture.
- Avoid excessive swinging or jerking actions by engaging the relevant muscles.
- Avoid rapid or abrupt motions by using a moderate and continuous range of motion.
- Exhale appropriately during the effort phase and inhale properly during the relaxation phase.
- If you're new to weight training, get the advice of a trained fitness expert to ensure you acquire the proper form and technique for each exercise.

The Value of Warm-up and Cool-down

Warming up properly is vital before beginning a weight training session. A warm-up gets the body ready for an exercise by boosting blood flow to the muscles, enhancing flexibility, and elevating core body temperature. This can be accomplished by dynamic stretching, mild aerobic activities, or a few warm-up sets with lesser weights. Similarly, a cool-down session following weight training is essential for recuperation and preventing muscular pain. It allows your heart rate and breathing to gradually return to normal and aids in the removal of waste products from your muscles, such as lactic acid. Static stretching, foam rolling, or modest cardiovascular activity can all be used as cool-down exercises.

Recovery and Rest

Rest and recuperation are just as vital in weight training as the sessions themselves. Muscles mend and develop stronger throughout the rest times. Overtraining without adequate recovery time can result in tiredness, poor performance, and an increased risk of injury. Make sure to include rest days in your weight training plan. Your muscles now have the ability to repair and adapt to the stress of training. Additionally, sleep and an adequate diet should be prioritized because they play an important part in the recuperation process.

CHAPTER 4. Routine for Full-Body Workouts

Introduction to Full-Body Workouts

A full-body exercise plan is an effective technique to train all main muscle groups at once. It's especially useful for people who are short on time or want to improve their general strength and muscular growth. Compound exercises that activate multiple muscle groups at the same time are common in full-body workouts.

Full-Body Workout Plan Example

Here's an example of a full-body training routine that may be done two to three times each week:

- **Squats:** three sets of ten repetitions
- Bench Press: three sets of ten repetitions
- 3 sets of 10 repetitions of bent-over rows
- **Lunges:** two sets of 12 repetitions each.
- Lat 2 sets of 12 repetitions of pulldowns
- 2 sets of 12 repetitions of bicep curls
- **Tricep Dips:** two sets of twelve reps
- 2 sets of 15 repetitions of calf raises

Remember to begin with a weight that will push you while also allowing you to retain appropriate technique. Gradually increase the weight or the number of sets and repetitions as you develop.

Progression and Intensification

To keep making progress in your full-body workout program, progressively raise the intensity. This can be accomplished by raising the weight of the exercises, increasing the number of sets and repetitions, or shortening the rest times between sets. You may also integrate variants of the exercises or use advanced training techniques like supersets, drop sets, or pyramids. These techniques assist to push your muscles in new ways, stimulating further growth and strength increases. However, it is critical to listen to your body and avoid pushing yourself too far. Gradual advancement is essential for preventing injuries and maintaining long-term growth.

Finally, knowing the fundamentals of weight training, such as different exercise kinds, good technique, warm-up and cool-down routines, and the significance of rest and recovery, is critical for a successful and safe training trip.Implementing a well-rounded full-body exercise plan and progressively increasing the intensity can assist you in meeting your fitness objectives and living a healthy lifestyle.

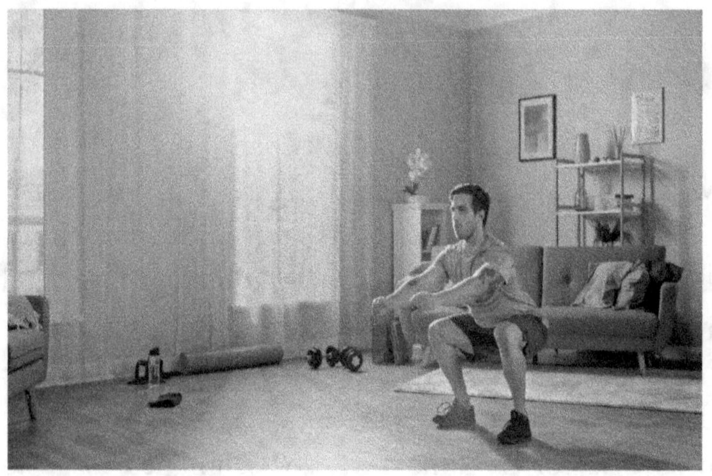

CHAPTER 5. Workouts for Specific Muscle Groups

Triceps and Chest

Focusing on the chest and triceps is vital for developing a strong upper body. These muscle groups are crucial for upper-body strength and stability and play an important part in different pushing activities. A chest and triceps exercise will help you build a well-rounded body and increase your overall strength. In order to successfully train the chest and triceps, you must include movements like bench presses, push-ups, chest flies, tricep dips, and tricep pushdowns into your regimen. These workouts work your chest and triceps muscles, creating development and definition.

To optimize benefits and limit the chance of injury, remember to do each exercise with perfect form and technique. To achieve balanced growth, combine complex workouts that include numerous muscle groups with isolation exercises that target particular muscles.

Biceps and Back

Maintaining appropriate posture, enhancing pulling actions, and developing an aesthetically attractive body all need a strong back and biceps. A tailored back and biceps exercise will help you increase strength and produce a well-proportioned upper body.

Include pull-ups, rows, lat pulldowns, deadlifts, and bicep curls in your regimen to properly train these muscular groups. These workouts target your back and biceps muscles, boosting development, strength, and definition.

To minimize muscle imbalances, it's critical to balance your workouts by include both pulling and pushing movements. Proper form and technique are essential for getting the most out of each workout and avoiding injury.

Shoulders and Legs

Strengthening your legs and shoulders not only improves your aesthetic look but also your general athleticism and functional strength. Specific exercises that target these muscle groups may help you acquire lower-body strength, stability, and upper-body mobility.

Include squats, lunges, leg presses, shoulder presses, lateral lifts, and upright rows in your regimen to properly train your legs and shoulders. These exercises target your leg and shoulder muscles, increasing development, strength, and stability.

You maximize benefits and reduce the chance of injury, make sure you complete these exercises with perfect form and technique. To guarantee complete development of these muscular groups, consider both complex exercises like squats and shoulder presses as well as isolation exercises like lateral raises.

Muscles of the Core and Abdomen

The cornerstone for total strength, stability, and balance is a strong core. Working out your core and abdominal muscles not only helps you get a toned stomach, but it also improves your posture and supports your spine.

Planks, crunches, Russian twists, bicycle crunches, and leg raises are excellent workouts for strengthening your core and abdominal muscles. These exercises strengthen and stabilize your core muscles, such as the rectus abdominis, obliques, and transverse abdominis.

To efficiently stimulate the targeted muscles and avoid strain or injury, it is essential to maintain good form and technique throughout these exercises. Consider integrating workouts that engage your complete core rather than just the rectus abdominis (the "six-pack" muscle) for overall core strength.

CHAPTER 6. Cardiovascular Workouts

Cardiovascular Training Advantages

Cardiovascular workouts, commonly known as cardio or aerobic exercises, provide significant health and well-being advantages. Regular aerobic exercise may enhance cardiovascular fitness, endurance, energy levels, and assist in weight control.

Cardiovascular activities stimulate the heart and lungs, improving their ability to transport oxygen and nutrients throughout the body. This improved efficiency improves overall cardiovascular health and lowers the risk of heart disease, hypertension, and other cardiovascular disorders.

Regular cardiac exercise also aids in weight reduction by improving metabolism and burning calories. It aids in the creation of a calorie deficit, which is necessary for losing extra body fat. Furthermore, cardio workouts produce endorphins, which may improve mood and decrease tension and anxiety.

Including Cardio in Your Routine

Cardiovascular workouts must be included in your fitness program for a well-rounded fitness plan. Depending on your tastes and fitness objectives, there are many methods to include cardio exercise into your routines.

Running, cycling, swimming, brisk walking, dancing, and utilizing cardio devices such as treadmills, ellipticals, or stationary cycles are all popular kinds of cardio exercise. Select activities that you love and that are appropriate for your fitness level and physical capabilities.

Aim for at least 150 minutes of moderate-intensity cardio or 75 minutes of vigorous-intensity cardio each week to properly include cardio into your routine, as advised by the American Heart Association. Begin with shorter workouts and progressively increase the length and intensity as your fitness level increases.

HIIT vs. Static Cardio

High-intensity interval training (HIIT) and steady-state cardio are two prominent cardiovascular training approaches. Both systems have merits, and which one is best for you depends on your fitness objectives and personal preferences.

HIIT incorporates periods of high-intensity activity followed by periods of rest or low-intensity recuperation. It is well-known for its time efficiency and capacity to burn a large number of calories in a short length of time. HIIT exercises may be hard and difficult, requiring maximal effort during high-intensity periods.

In contrast, steady-state cardio entails sustaining a continuous moderate-intensity effort over a sustained length of time. This style of aerobic exercise is lower in intensity yet allows for longer sessions. Individuals who like a steady pace and wish to gradually increase endurance frequently favor steady-state cardio. Both HIIT and steady-state cardio offer advantages, and a mix of the two may be included into your regimen to get the best results. HIIT may be an excellent way to improve cardiovascular fitness, enhance metabolism, and burn calories in a shorter amount of time. Steady-state cardio, on the other hand, is beneficial for endurance training and provides a low-impact choice for recuperation or longer-duration workouts.

Finally, adding specific muscle group training and cardiovascular exercises into your fitness program will help you gain general strength, stability, and better cardiovascular health. You may achieve your fitness objectives and improve your overall well-being by creating a balanced workout plan that includes workouts for various muscle groups as well as frequent aerobic training.

CHAPTER 7. Flexibility and stretching

The Value of Stretching

Stretching is an important part of any well-rounded exercise regimen. It involves the intentional lengthening of muscles, tendons, and other soft tissues in order to increase flexibility and range of motion. Stretching exercises, although frequently disregarded, may provide several advantages to your workout plan.

Stretching, for starters, aids with flexibility. Our muscles naturally tighten as we age, resulting in a reduced range of motion. Stretching on a regular basis helps to prevent this process by extending and releasing the muscles, allowing for increased flexibility and performance in physical activities.

Second, stretching may aid in the prevention of injuries. Stretching prepares the body for the rigors of exercise by improving flexibility and lowering the risk of muscle strains, tears, and joint problems. It also encourages improved posture and alignment, reducing the likelihood of developing muscle imbalances or postural disorders.

Third, stretching promotes muscle healing and relieves muscular pain. Stretching exercises help clear out lactic acid and other metabolic byproducts after a workout, decreasing muscular stiffness and facilitating speedier recovery. Stretching also increases blood circulation, which provides oxygen and nutrients to the muscles and assists in their repair.

Stretches of Various Types

Stretches come in a variety of forms, each targeting a certain muscle area and fulfilling a specific function.

Here are a few examples of frequent stretches:

- Static stretching is holding a stretch in a comfortable posture for an extended amount of time, generally about 30 seconds. It aids in progressively lengthening muscles and increasing flexibility.
- Dynamic stretching entails continuous movement over the whole range of motion. They are often used before to exercises to warm up the muscles and prepare them for physical activity.

- Proprioceptive Neuromuscular Facilitation (PNF) Stretching, PNF stretching includes contracting and releasing muscles to increase flexibility. It is often done with a partner and is very useful for developing range of motion.
- Active stretching is conducted without the need of any external support or equipment. They are performed by contracting opposing muscle groups while stretching the target muscle.
- Passive stretching entails employing an external aid, such as a partner, a strap, or gravity, to produce a deeper stretch. It increases range of motion by overcoming the body's inherent resistance.

Beginner Stretching Routine

If you're new to stretching, begin softly and gradually increase the intensity and length of your stretches.

A basic stretching practice for beginners is as follows:

- Stretch your neck by gently tilting your head to the right, bringing your right ear closer to your right shoulder. Do this for 10-20 seconds before changing to the other side. Complete 2-3 sets on each side.

- Shoulder Rolls, for 10-15 seconds, roll your shoulders forward in a circular motion, then reverse the direction. Make 2-3 sets.
- Sit on the floor with one leg straight out in front of you and the other bent with the sole of the foot on the inner thigh. Lean forward from your hips and grasp towards your toes. Do this for 10-20 seconds before s
- changing to the other side. Complete 2-3 sets on each side.
- Stretch your quadriceps by standing tall and holding onto a wall or a chair for support. Bend one knee and move your foot toward your glutes, grasping the ankle with your hand. Pull your foot closer to your glutes until you feel a stretch at the front of your thigh. Do this for 10-20 seconds before changing to the other side. Complete 2-3 sets on each side.
- Lean forward, hands on the wall, and maintain your rear leg straight. Your calf muscle should be stretched. Do this for 10-20

seconds before changing to the other side. Complete 2-3 sets on each side.

It's critical to listen to your body and prevent overstretching or bouncing, which might result in damage. You may progressively increase the time and intensity of your stretches as you feel more comfortable.

CHAPTER 8. Understanding Macronutrients in Nutrition and Diet

Macronutrients are the three major dietary components: carbohydrates, proteins, and fats. Each macronutrient has a distinct dietary guideline and plays an important function in the body.

- Carbohydrates, which are found in meals such as grains, fruits, vegetables, and legumes, supply energy to the body. Choose complex carbs, such as whole grains, which are high in fiber and give lasting energy.
- Proteins are required for tissue construction and repair, immunological function, and the production of enzymes and hormones. Protein-rich foods include lean meats, poultry, fish, eggs, dairy products, legumes, and plant-based proteins such as tofu and tempeh.
- Fats are required for hormone synthesis, nutrition absorption, and as a concentrated source of energy. Choose healthy fats like avocados, almonds, seeds, olive oil, and fatty seafood like salmon.

Bodybuilders' Meal Planning

Bodybuilders have specific dietary requirements to promote muscular development and recuperation. **Here are some meal preparation ideas for bodybuilders:**

- Make sure you're getting enough protein: With each meal, aim for a protein-rich source, such as lean meats, fish, eggs, or plant-based proteins like lentils and tofu.
- Consume complex carbs such as whole grains, sweet potatoes, and quinoa to fuel strenuous exercises and restore glycogen reserves.
- Include sources of healthy fats such as avocados, nuts, seeds, and olive oil to boost hormone production and general wellness.
- Consume an abundance of fruits and vegetables. These include important vitamins, minerals, and antioxidants that promote general health and assist in recuperation.
- Maintain optimum hydration, assist digestion, and enhance performance by drinking lots of water throughout the day.

Supplements may help novices improve their fitness journey, but they should never be used in lieu of a well-balanced diet.

Consider the following supplements:

- **Protein derived from whey:** Whey protein, a popular option for muscle rehabilitation and development, may be ingested as a smoothie or added to meals.
- **Multivitamins:** A high-quality multivitamin supplement will help you address nutritional deficiencies in your diet.
- **Omega-3 fatty acids:** These are found in fish oil supplements as well as plant-based sources such as flaxseed oil, and they help with joint health, heart health, and inflammation reduction.
- **Creatine Monohydrate:** Known for its capacity to boost strength and power, creatine monohydrate is commonly utilized by sportsmen and weightlifters.

Remember, it's vital to check with a healthcare practitioner or registered dietitian before taking any new supplements, since they can give individualized recommendations based on your unique requirements and objectives. By including stretching into your training regimen and keeping a balanced diet, you may increase flexibility, minimize the chance of injury, promote muscle development, and maximize overall health and well-being.

CHAPTER 9. Monitoring Progress and Making Changes

The Importance of Keeping Track of Your Workouts

Keeping track of your exercises is an important part of any fitness regimen. Keeping track of your development, whether you're a novice or an experienced athlete, gives vital insights into your performance and allows you to make educated choices for advancement. You may create a clear baseline, set reasonable objectives, and track your progress over time by recording your exercises.

Tracking enables you to record and assess data such as the number of repetitions, sets, weights lifted, distances traveled, and time required to finish an activity. This information gives you objective feedback on your performance and enables you to spot trends, strengths, and flaws. By routinely tracking your workouts, you may celebrate your accomplishments, find areas for improvement, and remain encouraged by seeing your progress firsthand. Tracking your exercises also helps you retain consistency and responsibility. You may examine patterns and discover possible roadblocks to your development by maintaining a log of your training sessions. It also keeps you on track with your fitness routine, ensuring that you are exercising at the appropriate frequency, intensity, and length.

Body Composition Analysis

Measuring body composition entails more than just weighing yourself on a scale. It gives you a more complete picture of your bodily changes and growth. Body composition analysis is the process of determining the percentage of fat, muscle, bone, and other components in your body. It allows you to analyze if your training program is producing the desired results and adapt appropriately.

Body fat percentage measures, skinfold caliper testing, bioelectrical impedance analysis (BIA), dual-energy X-ray absorptiometry (DEXA), and air displacement plethysmography (ADP) are all common ways of determining body composition. These methods may assist you in monitoring changes in your body fat percentage, muscular mass, and general physique. By periodically analyzing your body composition, you can evaluate the efficiency of your training routine and make the necessary changes to meet your objectives.

Remember that body composition measures are just one part of progress monitoring. To have a thorough knowledge of your fitness journey, examine additional signs such as energy levels, general fitness, and subjective well-being.

Changing Your Workout Routine

As you log your exercises and assess your progress, you may come into instances where you need to make changes to your training schedule. Changing your regimen is essential for keeping your body challenged, avoiding plateaus, and optimizing outcomes. When making changes, it is important to consider many things, including your current fitness level, particular objectives, available time, and any limits or injuries. Modifying exercise choices, intensity, volume, frequency, or rest intervals are examples of adjustments. You may, for example, raise the weight lifted, adjust the number of sets and repetitions, add new exercises, or rearrange your sessions.

It is critical to approach changes cautiously and gradually. Making significant changes to your fitness routine may put you at danger of injury or overtraining. Instead, make little changes and evaluate their influence on your development. You may adapt your training program to meet your particular requirements and assure continuing progress toward your objectives by constantly monitoring your sessions and being open to alterations.

CHAPTER 10. Common Errors and Troubleshooting

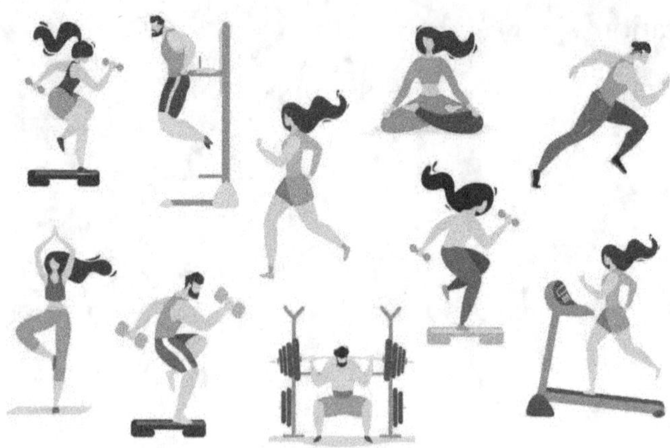

How to Avoid Common Pitfalls

Starting a fitness journey may be difficult, and it's important to be aware of typical mistakes that might stymie your progress.

Among the most prevalent errors are:

- Setting unreasonable objectives or expecting immediate results may lead to frustration and despair. Setting reasonable, attainable objectives is critical, as is understanding that fitness is a long-term commitment.

- Ignoring appropriate nutrition: Exercise alone is insufficient. Failure to nourish your body with a well-balanced diet might stifle your growth. Pay attention to your eating habits and make sure you're eating a well-balanced diet to help you reach your fitness objectives.

- Inconsistency in your training regimen: Inconsistency in your workout routine might stymie growth. Aim for frequent workout sessions and create a sustainable program that works for you.

- Overtraining, exercising too hard without enough rest and recuperation may result in tiredness, injury, and burnout. Listen to your body and include rest days in your training schedule.

Managing Plateaus

Plateaus are typical and annoying in any fitness endeavor. When you hit a plateau, it indicates that your body has acclimated to your present regimen and that development has temporarily paused.

- Change up your workouts by adding new exercises, changing the sequence of exercises, or varying the intensity and volume to push your body in new ways.
- Raise intensity, to break through the plateau, gradually raise the weights you lift, the pace of your cardio sessions, or the resistance in your exercises.
- Experiment with various training approaches. In order to shock your body and burst through the plateau, use diverse training strategies like as high-intensity interval training (HIIT), circuit training, or plyometrics.
- A brief period of rest and rehabilitation might sometimes help you break through a plateau. Allow your body to heal completely before resuming to your routines with fresh vigor.

Injury Prevention and Management

Injuries may be a setback in your fitness path, but they can frequently be avoided or treated properly. **Here are some pointers:**

- Warm up and cool down thoroughly before each exercise to prepare your muscles and joints. Similarly, to help with recuperation, cool down with stretching exercises.
- Exercise good form and technique. To limit the chance of injury, learn and practice proper form for each activity. If necessary, seek the advice of a trained fitness specialist.
- Gradually increase the intensity, volume, or weight of your workout. Gradual progression helps your body to adjust and reduces the likelihood of overuse issues.
- Pay attention to your body, keep an eye out for any pain or discomfort throughout your exercises. If you feel chronic discomfort, alter or discontinue the activity and, if required, see a healthcare practitioner.
- Cross-train, include a range of workouts and activities in your regimen to avoid overuse injuries and increase overall fitness.

Remember that safety should always come first. If you injure yourself, get medical treatment and follow the specified rehabilitation plan before returning to your exercises.

CONCLUSION

In conclusion, "Bodybuilding Workout Plan for Beginners" provides a thorough and well-structured instruction for individuals just starting out on their bodybuilding adventure. This book provides novices with the knowledge and resources they need to create a solid foundation of strength and muscle through straightforward instructions, progressive training routines, and a focus on appropriate form and technique. It fosters sustainable and healthy behaviors, assuring long-term success, by giving a balanced approach that involves both exercise and dietary counseling. Whether you're a total beginner or wanting to fine-tune your training regimen, this book is an excellent resource, allowing individuals to reach their bodybuilding objectives while putting their entire well-being first.

In addition, "Bodybuilding Workout Plan for Beginners" goes beyond just offering exercises and routines. It dives into basic bodybuilding concepts, emphasizing the necessity of increasing overload, rest and recovery, and the mind-muscle link. It helps readers avoid possible setbacks and optimize their success by tackling typical mistakes and misunderstandings. The engaging tone and user-friendly style of the book make it accessible to those with varied degrees of exercise knowledge. It simplifies complicated topics into easily consumable material, allowing newcomers to learn the essentials without becoming overwhelmed. The use of detailed pictures and step-by-step directions improves the learning experience, allowing readers to do exercises with confidence and precision.

Finally, "Bodybuilding Workout Plan for Beginners" emphasizes the importance of diet in attaining the best outcomes. It gives readers realistic information on macronutrient ratios, meal planning, and supplements, allowing them to fuel their bodies effectively and boost muscle growth. The book supports a healthy connection with food while discouraging severe or restrictive diets by highlighting the necessity of a balanced and sustainable approach to eating.